# Rheumatoid Arthritis

*The Hidden truth behind Rheumatoid Arthritis*

## Phillip K. Flood

# TABLE OF CONTENT

# INTRODUCTION

As the number of persons suffering from autoimmune disorders rises in the West, some research has linked these illnesses to male infertility, or the inability of men to conceive.

We know that joint problems can influence a woman's ability to conceive, but little is known about how it affects men. A study from 2021 suggested that men's infertility may be related to inflammatory arthritis, but further research is need to confirm this.

males with inflammatory joint diseases (IJDs) have higher birth rates than males without the condition, according to a recent study.
males with inflammatory joint diseases (IJDs) have higher birth rates than males without the condition, according to a recent study.

This recent study aimed to determine the number of children and the percentage of non-childbearing men with joint problems. 10,865 males from Norway who suffered from joint conditions such as psoriatic arthritis, spondyloarthritis, and rheumatoid arthritis were examined.

They were contrasted with 54,325 males who did not have these illnesses as a control group. Between 1967 and 2021, the 65,190 men in this group were responsible for the birth of 111,246 children.
The research separated births and childlessness into three time intervals (1967–85, 1986–99, and 2000–21), each of which corresponded to notable shifts in the use of medications to treat inflammatory joint illnesses.

According to the researchers' findings, males with IJDs often had more children throughout all time periods. The treatment of IJDs has undergone substantial changes in the most recent period, which made this more evident.

Examining the onset of the disease, the researchers discovered that males with IJDs who were diagnosed before the age of 20 or when they were fertile had comparable birth rates to those who did not have the condition. However, the groups with older diagnoses still included fewer childless men, indicating that variables other than the illness itself are important. Even if the study raises the possibility of a connection between joint disorders and fertility, it is important to note that it offers no convincing explanations for any of the observed phenomena.

The researchers observed that "Factors associated with developing or having an IJD might influence fertility, and this requires further investigation." In addition to the disease itself, factors outside the purview of this study may include emotional well-being, occupations, and smoking habits.
According to a study, men who have arthritis may have higher fertility than their friends who do not.

According to new research, men with inflammatory joint diseases, such rheumatoid arthritis, had a lower likelihood of being childless and a higher likelihood of having children than their counterparts in good health
The fact that Norwegian women with inflammatory joint disease have been documented to have reduced fertility gave the researchers the idea to examine males with the illness.

The researchers examined data on 10,865 Norwegian males with rheumatoid arthritis, psoriatic arthritis, or spondyloarthritis between 1967 and August 2021 in order to arrive at their findings, which were published in the Annals of the Rheumatic Diseases.

They chose to gauge fertility by looking at both the number of children and the absence of children.

The average number of children fathered by each patient was 1.8, as opposed to 1.7 in the comparison group, according to the data.

Approximately 20% of the patients were childless, while almost 40% of the comparison group did not have children.

While these variations persisted throughout time, the number of children with the biggest difference—an average of 1.8 vs 1.6—was found among those diagnosed after 2000.
With a risk of 22% compared to 28%, these patients likewise had the lowest chance of being childless.

The men diagnosed in their 30s had the biggest absolute difference in childlessness between 2000 and 21—22 percent against 32 percent.
It was discovered that the average age of first-time fatherhood was 28 in the comparison group and 27 in the males with inflammatory joint disease. According to these findings, men with arthritis do not only have normal fertility, but they also tend to have more children earlier in life. Dr. Gudrun David Sigmo of Stavanger University Hospital in Norway stated that male patients with inflammatory joint disease can feel reassured that their fertility will not be affected.

Substudies based on certain diagnoses, however, must to be carried out in order to provide patients with more specialized information.

"Our discovery of a lower risk of childlessness and a greater number of children per man in patients with inflammatory joint illness is new and leads to new theories about the relationships between immune-modulating medications, inflammatory rheumatic disorders, and fertility.

# CHAPTER ONE

## What you need to know about Rheumatoid arthritis

A persistent inflammatory condition that affects more than simply joints is rheumatoid arthritis. Some individuals may experience damage to many different body systems, including as the heart, blood vessels, lungs, skin, and eyes.

Rheumatoid arthritis is an autoimmune disease that happens when your body's immune system accidentally targets its own tissues.
In contrast to the gradual deterioration caused by osteoarthritis, rheumatoid arthritis damages the lining of your joints, resulting in excruciating swelling that may eventually lead to deformity and erosion of the bone.

Other bodily parts may also sustain harm from the inflammation linked to rheumatoid arthritis. Severe rheumatoid arthritis can still result in physical limitations, despite the fact that new drug alternatives have significantly improved treatment possibilities. Elements that could make you more susceptible to rheumatoid arthritis include:

Your intimate relations. Rheumatoid arthritis is more common in women than in men.
years old. Although rheumatoid arthritis can strike at any age, it usually first manifests in middle age.
Ancestry. You can be more susceptible to rheumatoid arthritis if a family member has the condition.
consuming tobacco. In particular, if you have a genetic predisposition to the condition, smoking raises your risk of developing rheumatoid arthritis. Additionally, it seems that smoking is linked to a higher severity of the disease.

Overweight. Obesity seems to be associated with a slightly increased risk of rheumatoid arthritis.

Your risk of developing: rises if you have rheumatoid arthritis.

bone weakening. Osteoporosis is a disorder that rheumatoid arthritis and some of the drugs used to treat it can increase your risk of developing a disorder that weakens your bones and increases the risk of fractures.

Nodules of rheumatism. Usually, these hard lumps of tissue form around pressure sites, like the elbows. But wherever in the body, including the heart and lungs, might develop these nodules.

mouth and eyes dry. A condition called Sjogren's syndrome, which lowers moisture levels in the lips and eyes, is far more common in those with rheumatoid arthritis.

illnesses. Both rheumatoid arthritis and many of the drugs used to treat it can weaken the immune system, which increases the risk of infections. Vaccinate yourself to protect against diseases including COVID-19, shingles, pneumonia, and influenza.

abnormal makeup of the body. Even in individuals with a normal body mass index (BMI), the ratio of fat to lean mass is frequently higher in rheumatoid arthritis patients.

carpal tunnel syndrome. When rheumatoid arthritis affects your wrists, the nerve that supplies most of your hand and fingers may be compressed by the inflammation.

cardiovascular issues. Artherosclerosis and inflammation of the sac enclosing your heart are two conditions that can be made worse by rheumatoid arthritis..

pulmonary illness. Breathlessness that worsens with time is more likely to occur in people with rheumatoid arthritis due to lung tissue inflammation and scarring.

Thyroid cancer. A type of blood tumors called lymphomas that arise in the lymphatic system are more common in people with rheumatoid arthritis.

The cause of rheumatoid arthritis (RA), a chronic systemic inflammatory illness, is uncertain. The hands and feet are most affected, and it typically manifests as bilateral symmetric polyarthritis (synovitis) (see the image below). On the other hand, extra-articular involvement of organs including the skin, heart, lungs, and eyes can be substantial in any joint that its lining, the synovial membrane.

 The development of RA is thought to occur when an external event (such as smoking cigarettes, contracting an infection, or experiencing trauma) causes an autoimmune reaction in a genetically predisposed person (e.g., a carrier of HLA-DR4 or HLA-DR1 [1]).

The primary target of RA is the joints, often several joints at once. Joints in the hands, wrists, and knees are frequently affected by RA. Damage to joint tissue results from inflammation of the joint lining in RA-affected joints. Deformity (misshapenness), unsteadiness (loss of balance), and chronic or persistent discomfort can all result from this tissue injury.


In addition to affecting other body parts, RA can also result in issues with organs like the heart, lungs, and eyes.
The following are possible extra characteristics of rheumatoid arthritis:

The tissue that covers the ends of the bones in a joint is damaged as a result of its effects on the joint lining.
RA frequently manifests symmetrically, which means that if one hand or knee is afflicted, the other hand or knee is frequently equally impacted.
The joints in the mouth, hands, elbows, shoulders, feet, spine, and knees can all be impacted.
RA can lead to fevers, exhaustion, and appetite loss.

In addition to the joints, the heart, lungs, blood, nerves, eyes, and skin can all experience health issues as a result of RA.
Fortunately, persons with the condition can enjoy productive lives thanks to current treatments.

## What is the course of rheumatoid arthritis?

The immune system's attack on joint tissues is unknown to doctors. But they are aware that rheumatoid arthritis can arise from a set of circumstances. Among the things that happen in this sequence are:

The development of RA is triggered by exposure to environmental conditions and a combination of genes.
Years before symptoms manifest, the immune system may be triggered. Although the autoimmune process can begin in other parts of the body, the effects of the immune system going awry usually concentrate in the joints. The synovium, which is the joint's inner lining, becomes inflamed due to immune cells.

A growth in cells, the synthesis of proteins, and other elements in the joint cause the synovium to thicken and cause chronic inflammation, which can cause pain, redness, and warmth.
As RA worsens, the inflammatory and swollen synovium presses harder into the joint, destroying the bone and cartilage inside.
The forces that cause the joint capsule to spread throughout the joint structure.
The tendons, ligaments, and surrounding muscles that stabilize and support the joint deteriorate over time and lose some of their functional strength. More discomfort, injury to the joint, and difficulties using the afflicted joint may result from this.

Rheumatoid arthritis complications
RA can be somewhat disabled since it gradually affects joints. Pain and issues with movement may result from it. Your ability to perform your regular daily routines and activities may be diminished. Additionally, this may result in issues like anxiety and despair.

The lungs, heart, skin, muscles, blood vessels, kidneys, nerves, and many other non-joint components of the body might also be impacted by RA. Death or serious disease may result from these complications.
.

# CHAPTER TWO

## Essential ways to know if one is infected with Rheumatoid arthritis

Rheumatoid arthritis symptoms and indicators could be as follows:

sore, heated, swollen joints
stiffness in the joints, which is typically worst in the mornings and after inactivity
lassitude, fever, and appetite decline
Early-stage rheumatoid arthritis usually affects smaller joints first, especially the joints connecting your toes and fingers to your foot.

The wrists, knees, ankles, elbows, hips, and shoulders are frequently affected as the illness worsens. The same joints on both sides of your body typically experience symptoms.

Rheumatoid arthritis patients also report having symptoms and indicators outside of their joints in about 40% of cases. The following areas could be impacted:
Skin Lungs Eyes
Kidneys and Heart
The salivary glands
neural tissue
skeletal system
Vascular structures
The severity and intermittent nature of rheumatoid arthritis symptoms can vary. There are intervals of relative remission, during which the pain and swelling lessen or stop, and intervals of heightened disease activity, known as flares. Rheumatoid arthritis can lead to deformities and displacements of joints with time.

A fever, malaise, arthralgias, weakness, and eventually joint inflammation and swelling are the most common early signs of RA in most people. The following are possible RA signs and symptoms:

Hand and foot symmetric polyarthritis (synovitis) with persistent onset (defining characteristic)
articular degradation that is progressive
engagement beyond the articulation
Having trouble completing daily living activities (ADLs)
constitutional signs and symptoms
The following issues ought to be covered during the physical exam:

Shoulders, wrists, elbows, and metacarpophalangeal joints are considered upper extremities.
Lower extremities: hips, knees, ankles, and feet
back of the neck
It's crucial to evaluate the following during the physical examination:
Hardness
sensitivity
ache when moving
Swelling irregularity
Motion limitation
Symptoms outside of the joints

One autoimmune condition is arthritis. Normally, the immune system aids in defending your body against illness and infection. Your body's defenses target the healthy tissue in your joints when you have rheumatoid arthritis. Medical issues pertaining to your heart, lungs, nerves, eyes, and skin may also result from it.

Although a hereditary component seems likely, doctors are unsure of what triggers this process. Rheumatoid arthritis is not primarily caused by genes, but it can be triggered by environmental factors such as bacterial or viral infections. Genes can also alter how the body responds to these triggers.

Using treat-to-target method, integrated approach comprising pharmacologic and nonpharmacologic medicines, and collaborative decision making, treatment of RA should be started early. The following tools can be used to help with treating to target:

RA disease activity measures were advised by the American College of Rheumatology (ACR) [2].
ACR/EULAR (European Alliance of Associations for Rheumatology) remission criteria [3]
Among the nonsurgical, nonpharmacologic treatments are the following:

Treatments using heat and cold
Braces and orthopaedics
exercise for therapy
In occupational therapy
Modest-sized apparatus
Cooperative safety instruction
Energy-saving instruction
The following groups have released pharmacologic therapy guidelines:

College of Rheumatology in America (2021) In [4]
The European Association of Rheumatology (2022) [5]
DMARDs, or nonbiologic disease-modifying antirheumatic medications, consist of the following:
Treatments using heat and cold
Braces and orthopaedics
exercise for therapy
In occupational therapy
Modest-sized apparatus
Cooperative safety instruction
Energy-saving instruction
The following groups have released pharmacologic therapy guidelines:

(2022) [5] European Alliance of Associations for Rheumatology

DMARDs, or nonbiologic disease-modifying antirheumatic medications, consist of the following:

Hydrochloroquine
Saline acetate Sulfasalazine
Leflunomide with Methotrexate
cyclosporin
golden salts
D-penicillamine
methylcycline
The following DMARDs are biologic tumor necrosis factor (TNF)-inhibiting:

Etanercept
inselimab
ADALIUMAB
The drug certolizumab
Golimumab Biologic non-TNF DMARDs consist of the subsequent:

Medication Rituximab
Akinra
Abatacept
Tacilizumab
The Sarilumab
Infliximab
bacitinib
Padacitinib
The following medications are also used therapeutically:

The corticosteroids
NSAIDs (nonsteroidal anti-inflammatory medications) Analgesics
Surgical interventions encompass the following:

The synovectomy
The Tenosynovectomy

realignment of tendon

Arthroplasty or reconstructive surgery

arthrodyses

For rheumatoid arthritis, which medication is the safest?

For rheumatoid arthritis, the safest medication is the one that offers the greatest therapeutic benefit with the fewest adverse effects. Your medical history and the intensity of your RA symptoms will determine how this changes. You and your healthcare provider will collaborate to create a treatment plan. The medications that your doctor recommends will depend on how bad your illness is.

Meeting with your healthcare physician on a regular basis is crucial. If required, they will adjust your treatment and monitor for any adverse effects. In order to assess the efficacy of your therapy and identify any potential adverse effects, your healthcare professional could prescribe certain tests.

Will my rheumatoid arthritis improve if I change my diet?

Dietary modifications may assist in lowering inflammation and other RA symptoms when paired with the therapies and drugs your doctor suggests. It won't heal you, though. Consult your physician about reducing processed carbs, salt, and harmful fats while increasing beneficial fats. Rheumatoid arthritis cannot be cured by natural remedies or nutritional supplements such as collagen. Under the guidance of your rheumatologist, these dietary modifications are both safer and more effective.

You can, however, alter your way of living to perhaps help with symptom relief. To lessen the strain on irritated joints, your rheumatologist might advise losing weight.

Additionally, rheumatoid arthritis patients are more likely to develop coronary artery disease. Dietary modifications may have an impact on high blood cholesterol, a risk factor for coronary artery disease. A nutritionist can advise on which foods to eat or stay away from in order to achieve a target cholesterol level.

Overview of Diagnosis and Tests

Numerous bodily systems are impacted by rheumatoid arthritis.

An autoimmune condition called rheumatoid arthritis affects multiple body systems.

Rheumatoid arthritis: what is it?

One chronic (continuous) autoimmune illness is rheumatoid arthritis (RA). It differs from other forms of arthritis in that it affects the joints on both sides of your body. Pain and inflammation symptoms could be present in your:

The fingers.
Hands.
Grasps
Knees
Ankles.
feet.
Toes.

The cartilage that often serves as a "shock absorber" in your joints is harmed by unchecked inflammation. This can eventually cause joint deformation. Your bone itself erodes with time. This may result in the fusion of your joint, which is your body's attempt to shield itself from ongoing discomfort.

Your body's defense against infections, or immune system, is aided in this process by certain cells. In addition to being produced in your joints, these chemicals circulate throughout your body and produce symptoms. Rheumatoid arthritis may occasionally affect areas of your body other than only your joints, such as your:

Heart, Lungs, Mouth, Skin, and Eyes.

Rheumatoid arthritis: who gets it?
In the US, around 1.3 million people suffer with rheumatoid arthritis. Individuals born with a gender identity are 2.5 times more likely to have it than those born with a gender identity.

What is the age of rheumatoid arthritis onset?
Between the ages of 30 and 60 is when RA typically first manifests. Rheumatoid arthritis, however, can strike anyone. It is known as young-onset rheumatoid arthritis (YORA) among children and young adults, who are typically between the ages of 16 and 40. It is known as later-onset rheumatoid arthritis (LORA) among those who get symptoms after the age of 60.

Signs and Origins
What signs of rheumatoid arthritis are present?
Everybody is affected by rheumatoid arthritis differently. Some persons experience joint pain over a period of years. For some, the symptoms of rheumatoid arthritis worsen quickly. Many persons experience flare-ups of symptoms followed by remissions of symptoms.

Rheumatoid arthritis symptoms include:

joint pain, edema, stiffness, and discomfort in multiple locations.
stiffness, particularly in the morning or after extended hours of sitting.
On both sides of your body, the same joints are painful and stiff.
weariness (severe exhaustion).
Weakness.
High temperature.
Does weariness arise from rheumatoid arthritis?

Each person with rheumatoid arthritis has a slightly different experience. However, a lot of RA sufferers claim that one of the hardest symptoms of their condition is weariness.

It is often very tiring to live with chronic pain. Additionally, it may be harder to manage your discomfort if you are tired. It is crucial to be aware of your body and to take pauses before you become very fatigued.

What are the signs of a flare-up of rheumatoid arthritis?
The signs of a flare-up of rheumatoid arthritis are similar to those of the disease itself. But there are ups and downs for RA sufferers. A flare-up occurs when you experience severe symptoms following a period of improved health. You'll probably have periods of improved health while receiving treatment.

Thereafter, a period of elevated disease activity is brought on by stress, climatic changes, particular foods, or infections.
 Flares can't always be avoided, but there are things you can do to help control them. Putting your symptoms and life events down in a notebook on a daily basis could be beneficial. To help you identify triggers, share this journal with your rheumatologist. You can then attempt to control those triggers.
What are rheumatoid arthritis's early warning signs?
Tiny joints, such as your fingers or toes, may feel tender or painful in the early stages of rheumatoid arthritis. You may also experience discomfort in a larger joint, such as your shoulder or knee.

These early symptoms of RA are comparable to a vibrating alarm clock. It might not have been sufficient every time to catch your eye. However, However, the early warning signals are crucial since therapy can start sooner if RA is identified. Prompt therapy can also reduce your risk of developing excruciating, long-lasting joint damage.

**How does early-stage rheumatoid arthritis manifest?**

For patients who have experienced rheumatoid arthritis symptoms for less than six months, providers may refer to their illness as "early rheumatoid arthritis."

Which four phases make up rheumatoid arthritis?
Stage1: The tissue surrounding your joint(s) is inflamed when rheumatoid arthritis is in its early stages. There can be some soreness and stiffness. They wouldn't notice harmful alterations in your bones if your doctor requested X-rays.
Stage 2: The inflammation has started to erode your joints' cartilage. A reduced range of motion and rigidity may be felt.
Stage 3: You have bone damage due to the extreme inflammation. More discomfort, stiffness, and decreased range of motion than in stage 2 are to be expected, along with some physical changes.
Stage 4: During this phase, your joints continue to deteriorate but the inflammation ends. Severe discomfort, edema, stiffness, and decreased movement will be experienced.

Your body is normally protected from disease by your immune system. Your immune system attacks your joints because of something when you have rheumatoid arthritis. Triggers include infections, smoking, and physical or psychological stress.

Does rheumatoid arthritis run in families?
Numerous genes that may be RA risk factors have been investigated by scientists. Your risk of rheumatoid arthritis is influenced by a few genetic differences as well as non-genetic factors. Factors that are not genetic include having sex and being among allergens and pollution.

Rheumatoid arthritis is more common in those who are born with variations in their human leukocyte antigen (HLA) genes. Your immune system can distinguish between proteins produced by your body and proteins from pathogens like bacteria and viruses with the aid of HLA genes.

Which conditions increase one's risk of getting rheumatoid arthritis?

The chance of getting rheumatoid arthritis is increased by multiple variables. Among these are:

Family history: Having a close relative with RA increases your risk of developing it yourself.
Sex: Rheumatoid arthritis is two to three times more common in women and those who are born with a female gender marker.
Smoking: Rheumatoid arthritis is exacerbated and an increased risk of the disease is associated with smoking.
Obesity: Being overweight increases the risk of RA development.

Diagnostics and Examinations
In what way is rheumatoid arthritis identified?
A rheumatologist, or doctor who specializes in treating arthritis, may be recommended to you by your healthcare provider. A number of variables are combined by rheumatologists to diagnose patients with rheumatoid arthritis.
  They will examine you physically and inquire about your symptoms and medical background. Your rheumatologist will prescribe imaging and blood testing.

The blood tests search for blood proteins, or antibodies, that indicate rheumatoid arthritis and inflammation. These might consist of:

Your joints' inflammation is confirmed by the erythrocyte sedimentation rate (ESR), also known as "sed rate."
protein C-reactive (CRP).
Approximately 80% of RA patients have positive rheumatoid factor (RF) tests.

Cyclic citrullinated peptides, or CCPs, are the target of antibodies in between 60% and 70% of rheumatoid arthritis patients.

Imaging tests may be recommended by your rheumatologist to check for indications that your joints are deteriorating.

The ends of the bones in your joints may deteriorate as a result of rheumatoid arthritis. Among the imaging tests that could be performed are:

Radiology images.
sound waves.
MRIs, or magnetic resonance imaging.
Sometimes a clear diagnosis of rheumatoid arthritis is made after a long period of observation by your healthcare practitioner.

# CHAPTER THREE

## Best way to prevent yourself from Rheumatoid arthritis.

What are the rheumatoid arthritis diagnostic criteria?
The symptoms, signs, and test findings your doctor looks for before diagnosing you with rheumatoid arthritis are known as diagnostic criteria. Years of study and clinical experience have formed their foundation. Not every RA patient meets every requirement. Nonetheless, rheumatoid arthritis is typically diagnosed using the following criteria:

arthritis due to inflammation in two or more big joints, such as the knees, ankles, hips, shoulders, and elbows.
arthritis causing inflammation in smaller joints.
Rheumatoid factor (RF) or CCP antibodies are examples of positive biomarker tests.
higher CRP values or a higher sedate onset rate.
You've experienced symptoms for more than six weeks.


Handling and Medical Interventions
What are the objectives of rheumatoid arthritis treatment?
Reducing joint discomfort and swelling is the main objective of rheumatoid arthritis treatment. By doing this, joint function ought to be preserved or enhanced. Treatment's long-term objective is to reduce or eliminate joint deterioration. Your quality of life is enhanced and your discomfort is decreased when joint inflammation is under control.

How does one treat rheumatoid arthritis?
It's crucial to visit your doctor as soon as you get symptoms because joint damage usually develops within the first two years of diagnosis. By treating

rheumatoid arthritis at this "window of opportunity," long-term effects may be avoided.

Rheumatoid arthritis is treated with a combination of medication, surgery, treatments, and lifestyle modifications. When choosing a course of action, your physician takes into account your age, overall health, past medical records, and severity of symptoms.

Which drugs are used to treat arthritis rheumatoid?
Using some medications early in treatment can help you have better results later on. Drug combinations seem to be just as safe as single-drug therapy, but they may also be more effective.

Numerous drugs can be used to prevent or delay the condition as well as to lessen joint pain, swelling, and inflammation. The following drugs are used to treat rheumatoid arthritis:

Anti-inflammatory non-steroidal medications (NSAIDs)
Anti-inflammatory medications that are non-steroidal reduce pain and inflammation. They consist of goods such as:

Advil®, Motrin®, and Ibuprofen.
Naproxen, often known as Aleve.
Aspirin.
COX-2 inhibitors

NSAIDs also include COX-2 inhibitors. Among them are goods like celecoxib (Celebrex®). Compared to conventional NSAIDs, COX-2 inhibitors have less gastrointestinal bleeding adverse effects.

The corticosteroids
Steroids, or corticosteroids, can also be used to treat inflammation and pain. Among them are cortisone and prednisone.

Antirheumatic medications that change disease (DMARDs)
In contrast to conventional NSAIDs, DMARDs alter your immune system to really slow down the progression of the illness. Both by themselves and in conjunction with steroids or other medications, your doctor may prescribe DMARDs. Common DMARDs consist of:

Trexall® has methotrexate.
Hydrochloroquine, also known as Plaquenil®.
Azulfidine® (sulfasalazine).
Leflunomide, better known as Rava.
Inhibitors of Janus kinase (JAK)


DMARDs also include JAK inhibitors. When methotrexate is insufficient to improve a patient's condition, rheumatologists frequently recommend JAK inhibitors. Among these goods are:

Meloxitinib (Xeljanz®) dosage.
Olumiant® Baracitinib.
biological substances
In the event that DMARDs are not well tolerated by you, your healthcare provider might recommend biologic response agents. Biologics target the chemicals that lead to joint inflammation. Providers believe biologics work better because they target the cells more precisely. Among these goods are:

Enbrel® (etanercept).
Rebikade®, or infliximab.
Take adalimumab (Humira®).
Anakirra (Kinaret®).
Orencia (Abatacept)®.
Rituxan®, also known as rituximab.
imimzia® (certolizumab).
Simponi® Golimumab.
Actemra® (tocilizumab).

In two to six weeks, biologics typically start to show results. Your doctor may prescribe them by itself or in addition to DMARDs like methotrexate.

For rheumatoid arthritis, which medication is the safest?
For rheumatoid arthritis, the safest medication is the one that offers the greatest therapeutic benefit with the fewest adverse effects. Your medical history and the intensity of your RA symptoms will determine how this changes. You and your healthcare provider will collaborate to create a treatment plan. The medications that your doctor recommends will depend on how bad your illness is.

Meeting with your healthcare physician on a regular basis is crucial. If required, they will adjust your treatment and monitor for any adverse effects. Your doctor could request certain tests to evaluate the efficacy of your  as well as any side effects you may have.

Will my rheumatoid arthritis improve if I change my diet?
Dietary modifications may assist in lowering inflammation and other RA symptoms when paired with the therapies and drugs your doctor suggests. It won't heal you, though. Consult your physician about reducing processed carbs, salt, and harmful fats while increasing beneficial fats. Rheumatoid arthritis cannot be cured by natural remedies or nutritional supplements such as collagen. Under the guidance of your rheumatologist, these dietary modifications are both safer and more effective.

ʹYou can, however, alter your way of living to perhaps help with symptom relief. To lessen the strain on irritated joints, your rheumatologist might advise losing weight.

Coronary artery disease is also more common in people with rheumatoid arthritis. Changes in nutrition can have an impact on high blood cholesterol, which is a risk factor for coronary artery disease. To achieve a desired cholesterol level, a nutritionist can suggest particular foods to eat or stay away from.

---

[1]

When does rheumatoid arthritis require surgery?
If a joint is seriously damaged, surgery might be the best option to restore function. If taking medicine doesn't relieve your discomfort, your doctor can potentially suggest surgery. RA-treating surgeries include:

Knee replacement.
Replacement of the hip.
further operations to fix a malformation.

For rheumatoid arthritis, what kinds of lifestyle modifications are helpful? It's normal to feel powerless over your quality of life when you have a chronic illness such as rheumatoid arthritis. Although there are elements of RA that are beyond your control, there are steps you can do to optimize your level of well-being.

Changes in lifestyle such as this include:

Take a nap
There is a significant chance that inflammatory joints could cause damage to surrounding soft tissue components, including ligaments and tendons. That's why you should give your swollen joints some rest. However, you should still make time for exercise. Keeping your joints well-ranged of motion and being physically healthy in general are crucial for managing RA.

Workout
Your gait may be slowed by pain and stiffness. Rheumatoid arthritis patients sometimes lose their ability to move. However, a lack of exercise can cause a person's muscles and joints to stiffen. Consequently, they decline increase in weariness and soreness as well as joint stability.

Exercise on a regular basis can help both avoid and counteract these consequences. If you want advice on safe exercise practices, you might want to start by visiting a physical or occupational therapist. Healthy exercise routines include:

range-of-motion exercises to protect and rebuild joint flexibility.
exercises aimed for improving strength.
Endurance-building exercises: walking, swimming, and cycling


Handling the rheumatism
Rheumatoid arthritis will never go away. But many individuals with the illness can go months or even years without experiencing flare-ups thanks to early identification and effective treatment. They can maintain regular employment and have fulfilling lives as a result.

The principal forms of treatment consist of:

Long-term medications that reduce symptoms and delay the condition's progression Supporting therapies, like physiotherapy and occupational therapy, to help you stay mobility and manage any issues you may be having with daily activities
surgical intervention to address any developing joint issues.

Printed in Great Britain
by Amazon

42580231R00020